Anti Inflammatory Diet: Detox Diet:

Weight Loss for Beginners & Detox Cleanse to Heal the Inflammation, Lose Belly Fat & Increase Energy

Emma Rose

Anti-Inflammatory Diet for Beginners

Lose Weight Fast, Optimize Health, Slow Aging, Fight Inflammation, Conquer Pain & Increase Energy with the Anti-Inflammation Diet Recipes

Emma Rose

Table of Contents

Introduction

I want to thank you and congratulate you for purchasing the book, "Anti-Inflammatory Diet for Beginners: Lose Weight Fast, Optimize Health, Slow Aging, Fight Inflammation, Conquer Pain & Increase Energy with the Anti-Inflammation Diet Recipes."

This book is a compilation of anti-inflammation recipes that will help you lose excess weight fast and slow the body's aging process so you will always feel at your best the whole day. These recipes are also recommended by professionals to fight inflammation to prevent any complications associated with this condition. Also, you can use these recipes to help boost your energy for optimal health.

In this book, you will find recipes for breakfast, lunch, dinner, and dessert that you can mix and match to design your own meal plan. Aside from being anti-inflammatory, these recipes can also be used for other special diets like paleo and gluten-free diet.

Thanks again for purchasing this book, I hope you enjoy it! Please take some time to stop by and LIKE our Facebook page:

https://www.facebook.com/joypublishing

With gratitude,

Emma Rose

Chapter 1: The Basics of The Anti-Inflammatory Diet

Chronic inflammation has been tagged as one of the root causes of severe illnesses including most cancers and heart attack. Inflammation is a natural reaction of the body when it needs to heal an infection or injury. However, when inflammation occurs for no particular reason, it destroys the body and eventually causes illness.

Chronic inflammation is caused by excessive exposure to toxins, stress, genetic predisposition, lack of exercise, and unhealthy diet. Since diet plays a big role in containing this condition, it is important to learn how to choose the right food to reduce the risk of diseases especially in the long-term.

The Anti-Inflammatory diet is not intended to help the person lose weight or to follow a strict diet plan. It is more of a guide to choose the right foods so the body stays in its optimal state. Aside from preventing inflammation, this diet also provides vitamins, dietary fiber, minerals, and other nutrients for steady energy.

General Tips for Anti-Inflammatory Diet

1. Try different varieties of food each meal.

2. Incorporate as much fresh foods into each meal.

3. Minimize consumption of fast food and processed food.

4. Eat vegetables and fruits every day.

5. Consume between 2,000 to 3,000 calories each day. If you are less active, you will need lesser calories.

6. 50% of your calorie intake should come from carbohydrates, 30% should come from fat and 20% should come from protein.

7. Drink more water or, if not, choose beverages that contain mostly water like fruit juices and tea.

8. Purify your drinking water.

Chapter 2: Breakfast Recipes

Cherry Quinoa Porridge

Ingredients:

- ✓ 1 cup of water
- ✓ ½ cup of dried unsweetened cherries
- ✓ ½ cup of dry quinoa
- ✓ ½ tsp of vanilla extract
- ✓ 1 tbsp of honey
- ✓ ¼ tsp of ground cinnamon

Procedure:

1. Prepare a medium-sized saucepan and set it over medium-high heat. Then, add in the water, dry quinoa, unsweetened cherries, vanilla extract, and ground cinnamon. Stir the ingredients together then bring the mixture to a boil.

2. Reduce the heat then place the lid on the saucepan. Let it simmer for 15 minutes or until the quinoa is tender and all the liquid has been absorbed.

3. Drizzle with honey then serve.

Raspberry Green Tea Smoothie

Ingredients:

- ✓ 1 ½ cups of chilled green tea
- ✓ 1 banana
- ✓ 2 cups of frozen raspberries (unsweetened)
- ✓ 1 tbsp of honey
- ✓ ¼ cup of protein powder

Procedure:

1. In a blender, add in the chilled green tea and honey. Combine the liquids together. Then, add in the banana, unsweetened raspberries, and protein powder. Blend until the mixture becomes smooth.

Gingerbread Oatmeal

Ingredients:

- ✓ 1 cup of water

- ✓ ¼ cup of dried and unsweetened cherries OR cranberries

- ✓ ½ cup of old-fashioned oats

- ✓ 1 tsp of ground ginger

- ✓ ¼ tsp of ground nutmeg

- ✓ ½ tsp of ground cinnamon

- ✓ 1 tbsp of flaxseeds

- ✓ 1 tbsp of molasses

Procedure:

1. Prepare a small saucepan and set it over medium-high heat. Add in the water, old-fashioned oats, unsweetened cherries or cranberries, ground ginger, ground cinnamon, and ground nutmeg. Stir the ingredients together. Bring the mixture to a boil then reduce the heat and simmer for 5 more minutes or until almost all of the liquid has been absorbed.

2. Add in the flaxseeds then cover the pan. Set it aside for 5 minutes.

3. Drizzle with molasses then serve.

Ginger Apple Muffins

Ingredients:

- ✓ 2 cups of all-purpose flour
- ✓ 1 tbsp of baking powder
- ✓ 2/3 cup of sugar
- ✓ ½ tsp of salt
- ✓ 1 tsp of ground ginger
- ✓ 1 tsp of ground cinnamon
- ✓ ¾ cup of unsweetened almond milk
- ✓ ½ cup of mashed ripe banana
- ✓ 1 cup of shredded apple
- ✓ 1 tbsp of apple cider vinegar
- ✓ ½ cup of finely chopped crystallized ginger

Procedure:

1. Turn on the oven and set it to 400F. Prepare a muffin pan with 12 cups and spray it with cooking spray or line it with paper liners.

2. In a large mixing bowl, add in the all-purpose flour, baking powder, sugar, ground cinnamon, salt, and ground ginger. Whisk the ingredients together until properly combined.

3. In a separate bowl, add in the unsweetened almond milk, apple, banana, apple cider vinegar, and crystallized ginger. Stir the ingredients together then gradually add in the flour mixture while stirring. Mix until the ingredients are well-incorporated. Fill the muffin cups with the batter about 2/3 of the way.

4. Place the muffin pan in the oven and bake for 15 minutes or until the muffins are done. To check, just insert a toothpick into the center of the muffin and, if it comes out clean,   you'll   know   it's   done.

Buckwheat and Quinoa Granola

Ingredients:

- ✓ 3 tbsp of honey
- ✓ 1 tsp of vanilla extract
- ✓ 3 tbsp of liquid coconut oil
- ✓ ¼ tsp of ground cinnamon
- ✓ 1 cup of buckwheat groats
- ✓ ¼ tsp of ground ginger
- ✓ 1 cup of cooked quinoa
- ✓ ½ cup of dried cranberries (unsweetened)
- ✓ ½ cup of old-fashioned oats

Procedure:

1. Turn on the oven and set it to 325F. Prepare a baking sheet and spray it with cooking spray or line it with parchment paper. You can also use a silicon baking mat if you have one.

2. In a bowl, add in the honey, liquid coconut oil, vanilla extract, ground cinnamon, and ground ginger. Stir the ingredients together until properly combined. In a larger bowl, add in the buckwheat groats, cooked quinoa, and old-fashioned oats. Stir then add in the honey mixture. Mix

until the ingredients are thoroughly combined. Spread the mixture onto the baking sheet and spread it evenly.

3. Place the baking sheet into the oven and bake for 40 minutes or until the grains are beginning to brown. Remove the pan from the oven then stir in the dried unsweetened cranberries. Place the baking sheet on a cooling rack and let it cool down completely before you store it in a tightly sealed container.

Spinach and Mushroom Frittata

Ingredients:

- ✓ 1 lb of button mushrooms, sliced
- ✓ 1 tbsp of freshly chopped garlic
- ✓ 1 large onion, chopped
- ✓ 1 lb of fresh spinach
- ✓ 6 large egg whites
- ✓ ¼ cup of water
- ✓ 4 large eggs
- ✓ ½ tsp of ground turmeric
- ✓ 5 oz of firm tofu
- ✓ ½ tsp of kosher salt
- ✓ ½ tsp of freshly cracked black pepper

Procedure:

1. Turn on the oven and set it to 350F.

2. Prepare a 10" ovenproof nonstick skillet or sauté pan and spray it with cooking oil. Set the pan over medium-high heat then sauté the mushrooms until they are golden brown. Add in the onion and cook for 3 minutes or until the onion is tender. Add in the garlic and cook for 30

seconds. Add in the water and spinach then place a lid on the pan. Cook for 2 minutes or until the spinach is wilted. Then, remove the lid and continue cooking until the liquid has completely evaporated.

3. In a blender, add in the egg whites, tofu, eggs, turmeric, black pepper, and salt. Process the ingredients until it forms a smooth mixture. When the liquid has completely evaporated from the pan, pour in the egg mixture to the spinach.

4. Remove the pan from the heat and transfer it into the oven. Bake for 25 minutes or until the eggs are set in the middle. Remove the pan from the oven and invert it on a serving plate to transfer the frittata and let stand for 10 minutes. Slice into wedges then serve.

Gluten-Free Strawberry Crepes

Ingredients:

- ✓ 6 cups of sliced strawberries
- ✓ 4 large eggs
- ✓ 2 tbsp of sugar OR honey
- ✓ 1 cup of unsweetened almond milk
- ✓ 1 tsp of vanilla extract
- ✓ 2 tbsp of light olive oil
- ✓ 1 tbsp of light brown sugar
- ✓ ¾ cup of gluten-free flour baking mix
- ✓ 1/8 tsp of salt

Procedure:

1. In a mixing bowl, combine the strawberries and sugar or honey. Let stand for 30 minutes at room temperature.

2. In a medium-sized bowl, add in the eggs, unsweetened almond milk, light olive oil, vanilla extract, light brown sugar, and salt. Whisk the ingredients together until well-incorporated. Then, add in the gluten-free flour baking mix. Continue whisking until the ingredients are properly combined.

3. Prepare an 8" nonstick skillet or crepe pan and set it over medium heat. Take ¼ cup of batter and add it into the pan. Swirl to coat the pan. Cook for 45 seconds or until the crepe is just beginning to brown. Flip and cook the other side for 10 seconds then transfer in onto a serving plate.

4. Place ½ cup of the strawberry mixture on half of the crepe then fold the crepe in half to form a semicircle. Drizzle syrup from the strawberry mixture over the crepe then serve.

Chapter 3: Lunch Recipes

Quick and Easy Pumpkin Soup

Ingredients:

- ✓ 1 cup of chopped onion
- ✓ 1 clove of garlic, minced
- ✓ 1 1" piece of gingerroot, peeled and minced
- ✓ 6 cups of vegetable stock, divided
- ✓ 1 tsp of salt
- ✓ 4 cups of pumpkin puree
- ✓ ½ tsp of fresh thyme, chopped
- ✓ 1 tsp of fresh parsley, chopped
- ✓ ½ cup of half-and-half

Procedure:

1. Prepare a large soup pot and set it over medium-high heat. Add in the onion, gingerroot, garlic, and ½ cup of vegetable stock into the pot and stir. Cook the vegetables for 5 minutes or until the vegetables are tender.

2. Add in the pumpkin puree, salt, thyme, and the remaining 5 ½ cups of vegetable stock. Stir the ingredients together and cook for 30 minutes.

3. Pour the soup in a food processor or use a handheld blender to puree the mixture until it becomes smooth.

4. Add in half-and-half into the soup and stir. Then, transfer the soup on a serving bowl and sprinkle with fresh parsley before serving.

Kippers Salad

Ingredients:

- ✓ ½ cup of reduced-fat mayonnaise
- ✓ 1 stalk of celery, finely chopped
- ✓ 1 small onion, finely chopped
- ✓ 1 tbsp of chopped fresh parsley
- ✓ 1 clove of garlic, minced
- ✓ 1 tsp of lemon juice
- ✓ 1/8 tsp of salt
- ✓ 1 (6 oz) can of kippers, drained
- ✓ 1/8 tsp of ground black pepper

Procedure:

1. In a mixing bowl, add in the mayonnaise, onion, celery, parsley, lemon juice, garlic, salt, and black pepper. Stir the ingredients together until well-incorporated. Add in the kippers and gently mix to combine. Place it inside the refrigerator until ready to use.

Roasted Chicken Wraps

Ingredients:

- ✓ ½ cup of reduced-fat mayonnaise
- ✓ 1 tsp of freshly cracked black pepper
- ✓ 2 tbsp of pickle juice
- ✓ 1 ½ cups of shredded red cabbage
- ✓ ¼ tsp of kosher salt
- ✓ 1 tbsp of apple cider vinegar
- ✓ ¼ tsp of cayenne pepper
- ✓ 6 whole wheat OR mixed grain flatbreads
- ✓ 1 deli-roasted chicken, cooled

Procedure:

1. In a large bowl, add in the mayonnaise, black pepper, and pickle juice. Stir the ingredients together until well-combined then place the bowl in the refrigerator. In another bowl, add in the red cabbage, salt, apple cider vinegar, and cayenne pepper. Toss the ingredients to combine.

2. Remove and throw away the bones and skin from the chicken then shred the meat to make bite-sized pieces. Add

the chicken pieces into the mayonnaise mixture and mix thoroughly.

3. Divide the chicken mixture and the cabbage mixture evenly among the slices of flatbreads. Roll to secure the filling and enjoy.

Persimmon and Pear Salad

Ingredients:

- ✓ 1 tsp of whole grain mustard
- ✓ 3 tbsp of extra virgin olive oil
- ✓ 2 tbsp of fresh lemon juice
- ✓ 1 shallot, minced
- ✓ 1 ripe persimmon, sliced
- ✓ 1 tsp of minced garlic
- ✓ 1 ripe red pear, sliced
- ✓ 6 cups of baby spinach
- ✓ ½ cup of chopped pecans, toasted

Procedure:

1. In a salad bowl, add in the whole grain mustard, lemon juice, olive oil, shallot, and garlic. Whisk the ingredients together until well-incorporated. Add in the persimmon, red pear, pecans, and baby spinach then toss to coat. Serve immediately.

Roasted Sweet Potato Soup

Ingredients:

- ✓ 2 ½ lbs of sweet potatoes
- ✓ ¼ tsp of kosher salt
- ✓ 1 tbsp of extra virgin olive oil
- ✓ ½ tsp of freshly cracked pepper
- ✓ 1 1" piece of ginger, peeled and minced
- ✓ 1 ½ cups of thinly sliced leeks OR onions
- ✓ 1 tsp of minced garlic
- ✓ 1 tsp of chopped fresh thyme leaves
- ✓ ½ cup of dry white wine
- ✓ 5 cups of vegetable broth
- ✓ 2 cups of orange juice

Procedure:

1. Turn on the oven and set it to 400F.

2. Remove the skins from the sweet potatoes and cut it into 1" pieces. Prepare a baking sheet and place the potatoes on it. Drizzle with olive oil and season using salt and pepper. Place the baking sheet in the oven and bake for 45 minutes

23

or until the sweet potatoes are well-browned and tender. Toss occasionally.

3. Prepare a large soup pot or Dutch oven and spray it with cooking spray. Set it over medium-high heat. Add in the leeks and cook for 8 minutes or until the leaves are tender and wilted. Add in the garlic and ginger and cook for 1 minute. Add in the dry white wine. Stir then bring the mixture to a boil. Continue cooking until the white wine has completely evaporated then add in the vegetable broth. Add in the thyme and sweet potatoes. Stir and bring the soup to a boil. Turn down the heat and simmer for 20 minutes or until all the vegetables are tender.

4. Pour the soup in an immersion blender and puree until it becomes smooth. Heat the soup again before serving.

Smoked Trout Tartine

Ingredients:

- ✓ 2 tbsp of freshly squeezed lemon juice

- ✓ 1 tsp of Dijon mustard

- ✓ 1 tbsp of extra virgin olive oil

- ✓ A pinch of sugar

- ✓ 2 tbsp of capers, rinsed and drained

- ✓ ¾ lb of smoked trout, flaked into bite-size pieces

- ✓ ½ cup of roasted red peppers, diced

- ✓ 1 stalk of celery, finely chopped

- ✓ ½ (15 oz) can of cannellini beans, drained and rinsed

- ✓ 2 tbsp of minced onion

- ✓ 4 large ½" thick slices of crusty whole grain bread, toasted

- ✓ 1 tsp of chopped fresh dill

- ✓ Dill sprigs

Procedure:

1. In a large bowl, add in the lemon juice, olive oil, Dijon mustard, and sugar. Whisk the ingredients together. Add in

the trout, capers, red peppers, cannellini beans, celery, onion, and dill. Toss the ingredients to combine.

2. Arrange the bread slices on a serving plate. Divide the trout mixture equally among the bread slices then place the mixture on top of the bread. Use the dill sprigs for garnish then   serve.

Lentil and Garbanzo Soup

Ingredients:

- ✓ 2 onions, chopped
- ✓ 1 cup of diced carrots
- ✓ 1 cup of chopped celery
- ✓ 2 tsp of grated fresh ginger
- ✓ 1 tsp of garam masala
- ✓ 1 tsp of minced garlic
- ✓ 1 tsp of turmeric
- ✓ ¼ tsp of ground cayenne pepper
- ✓ ½ tsp of ground cumin
- ✓ 6 cups of vegetable broth OR stock
- ✓ 2 (15 oz) cans of garbanzo beans, rinsed and drained
- ✓ 1 cup of lentils
- ✓ 1 (14.5 oz) can of petit diced tomatoes, undrained

Procedure:

1. Prepare a large soup pot and spray it with cooking spray. Set it over medium-high heat. Add in the onions and sauté for 3 minutes or until the onions are tender.

2. Add in the celery and carrots then cook for another 5 minutes.

3. Add in the garlic, garam masala, turmeric, cumin, and cayenne pepper. Stir and cook for 30 seconds.

4. Pour in the vegetable broth or stock and add in the lentils, garbanzo beans, and tomatoes. Stir and cook for 90 minutes or until the lentils become tender.

5. To make the soup a bit creamier and thicker, you can puree half of it and stir it back into the pot.

Chapter 4: Dinner Recipes

Poached Eggs with Curried Vegetables

Ingredients:

- ✓ 2 tsp of extra virgin olive oil
- ✓ 2 cloves of garlic, minced
- ✓ 1 large onion, chopped
- ✓ 1 tbsp of yellow curry powder
- ✓ 2 medium zucchinis, diced
- ✓ ½ lb of sliced button mushrooms
- ✓ 1 (14 oz) can of chickpeas, drained
- ✓ 1/8 tsp of crushed red pepper
- ✓ 1 cup of water
- ✓ ½ tsp of white vinegar
- ✓ 4 large eggs

Procedure:

1. Prepare a large nonstick skillet and set it over medium-high heat. Add in the onion and sauté for 4 minutes or until the onion is tender. Add in the garlic and cook for 30 seconds. Add in the curry powder and stir the ingredients together. Cook for 1 minute or until the mixture is very fragrant.

2. Add in the mushrooms and cook for 5 minutes or until the mushrooms are tender and have released all of its liquid. Add in the chickpeas, zucchini, red pepper, and water. Stir then bring the liquid to a boil. Turn down the heat and place a lid over the pan. Let it simmer for 15 minutes or until the zucchini becomes tender.

3. Prepare a large saucepan and fill it with water about 3" deep. Let it boil then turn the heat down. Add in the white vinegar and let it simmer.

4. Crack the eggs then gently slip it into the simmering liquid one at a time. Then, cook for 3 minutes or until the eggs are cooked according to your desired doneness. Remove the eggs from the hot water using a slotted spoon.

Weeknight Turkey Chili

Ingredients:

- ✓ Vegetable cooking spray
- ✓ 1 tbsp of garlic, minced
- ✓ 1 large onion, chopped
- ✓ 1 ½ lbs of ground turkey
- ✓ 1 (28 oz) can of crushed tomatoes
- ✓ 2 cups of water
- ✓ 1 (16 oz) can of kidney beans, drain then rinse
- ✓ 2 tsp of turmeric
- ✓ 2 tbsp of chili powder
- ✓ 1 tsp of smoked paprika
- ✓ 1 tsp of ground cumin
- ✓ 1 tsp of dried oregano
- ✓ 1 tsp of hot sauce

Procedure:

1. Prepare a large soup pot and spray it with vegetable cooking spray. Add in the onion and cook for 5 minutes or until the onion becomes tender and starts to brown. Add in

the garlic and cook for 30 seconds. Add in the ground turkey and cook for 10 minutes. Stir the ingredients frequently. Add in the water, tomatoes, kidney beans, chili powder, turmeric, paprika, oregano, cumin, and hot sauce. Stir the ingredients together then bring the mixture to a boil.

2. Turn the heat down and let it simmer for 30 minutes

3. .

Crusted Tilapia with Kale

Ingredients:

- ✓ ¼ cup of roasted Brazil nuts
- ✓ 2 tbsp of grated parmesan cheese
- ✓ ½ cup of fresh bread crumbs
- ✓ ¼ cup of whole grain mustard
- ✓ Vegetable cooking spray
- ✓ 1 ½ lbs of tilapia fillets
- ✓ 1 tbsp of sesame oil
- ✓ 1 ½ heads of kale, chopped
- ✓ 1 clove of garlic, mashed
- ✓ ¼ tsp of kosher salt
- ✓ 2 tbsp of toasted sesame seeds

Procedure:

1. Turn on the oven and set it to 400F. Prepare a baking sheet and spray it with vegetable cooking spray.

2. In a food processor, add in the Brazil nuts and process until the nuts are ground finely. In a small bowl, add in the ground nuts, parmesan cheese, and breadcrumbs. Stir the ingredients together until properly combined.

3. Place the tilapia fillets on the prepared baking sheet. Spread the mustard evenly on top of the fish fillets. Divide the breadcrumb mixture evenly among the fillets of fish. Spray the fish fillets with vegetable cooking spray. Place the baking pan into the oven and bake for 8 minutes or until the fish is properly cooked.

4. Prepare a large stainless steel or cast-iron skillet and set it over medium-high heat. Add in the sesame oil and wait for 15 seconds before adding in the garlic. Cook for 20 seconds then add in the kale. Cook for 7 minutes or until the kale becomes tender. Stir frequently while cooking. Add in the sesame seeds and toss the ingredients to combine.

5. Serve the fish fillets with kale on the side.

Red Pepper and Turkey Pasta

Ingredients:

- ✓ 3 large red bell peppers

- ✓ 1 large onion, chopped

- ✓ 3 tbsp of extra virgin olive oil

- ✓ 2 tsp of minced garlic

- ✓ 1 tbsp of red wine vinegar

- ✓ 2 tbsp of fresh oregano, chopped

- ✓ 2 lbs of ground turkey

- ✓ 2 lbs of cooked rigatoni

Procedure:

1. Cut the bell peppers in half. Remove the membranes and seeds then chop the peppers coarsely.

2. Prepare a Dutch oven and set it over medium heat. Add in the olive oil. Wait until the oil is hot before adding in the red bell peppers and onion. Cook for 20 minutes or until the peppers become very tender. Add in the garlic and cook for another 5 minutes.

3. Pour the mixture in a food processor or blender and process until it becomes smooth. Then, return the sauce into the pan and set it over medium-low heat. Add in the

red wine vinegar and oregano. Stir and taste. Adjust the seasonings if needed.

4. Prepare a large skillet and spray it with vegetable cooking spray. Add in the ground turkey and sauté until cooked and beginning to brown. Add in the turkey into the sauce and let it simmer for 20 minutes.

5. Place the rigatoni on a serving dish then pour the sauce over the pasta. Serve while still hot.

Steamed Salmon with Zucchini

Ingredients:

- ✓ 1 onion, thinly sliced
- ✓ 2 small zucchini, thinly sliced
- ✓ 1 lemon, thinly sliced
- ✓ 1 cup of white wine
- ✓ 4 (6 oz) fillets of salmon
- ✓ ½ cup of water
- ✓ ¼ tsp of kosher salt
- ✓ ¼ tsp of freshly ground pepper

Procedure:

1. Prepare a large Dutch oven then add in the onion, lemon, zucchini, white wine, and water.

2. Take the salmon fillets and season it using the kosher salt and freshly ground pepper. Place a steamer rack over the vegetables in the Dutch oven. Spray the rack with cooking spray. Set the Dutch oven over medium-high heat and wait for the liquid to boil.

3. Adjust the heat to medium-low and place the salmon fillets on the steamer rack. Place a lid over the Dutch oven and steam for 8 minutes or until the fillets are cooked through.

4. Remove the fish from the steamer rack and transfer the contents of the Dutch oven on a serving platter. Place the fish fillets on top of the vegetables then serve.

Black Bean and Sweet Potato Burgers with Lime Mayonnaise

Ingredients:

- ✓ ½ cup of reduced fat mayonnaise
- ✓ ½ tsp of hot sauce
- ✓ 1 lime
- ✓ Vegetable cooking spray
- ✓ 1 jalapeno, minced
- ✓ 1 small onion, chopped
- ✓ 2 tsp of ground cumin
- ✓ 2 (14.5 oz) cans of black beans, drain then rinse and mash
- ✓ 2 tsp of minced garlic
- ✓ 2 cups of grated raw sweet potato
- ✓ 1 cup of plain breadcrumbs, divided
- ✓ 1 egg, lightly beaten
- ✓ Whole wheat hamburger buns

Procedure:

1. Turn on the broiler and set it to medium-high heat. Place an oven rack about 4" to 5" from the broiler.

2. Take the zest and juice from the lime and add it into a small bowl. Add in the hot sauce and mayonnaise. Stir the ingredients together until properly combined then place the bowl in the refrigerator until needed.

3. Prepare a large skillet and set it over medium-high heat. Spray it with cooking spray then add in the onion. Cook for 4 minutes or until the onion is tender. Add in the jalapeno, garlic, and cumin. Cook for 30 seconds while stirring.

4. Transfer the onion mixture into a large bowl. Add in the sweet potato, black beans, ½ cup of breadcrumbs, and egg. Stir the ingredients together until well-combined.

5. Form the breadcrumb mixture into 8 patties and sprinkle each with the remaining breadcrumbs. Prepare a baking sheet and spray it with cooking spray. Arrange the patties on the baking sheet and spray with cooking spray.

6. Place the baking sheet into the oven and broil each side for 8 minutes or until the patties are cooked through and golden brown in color. Serve on hamburger buns with the mayonnaise mixture.

Quinoa and Turkey Stuffed Pepper

Ingredients:

- ✓ 1 cup of uncooked quinoa

- ✓ ½ tsp of salt

- ✓ 2 cups of water

- ✓ ½ lb of fully-cooked smoked turkey sausage, already diced

- ✓ ¼ cup of extra virgin olive oil

- ✓ ½ cup of chicken stock

- ✓ 3 tbsp of chopped pecans, toasted

- ✓ 2 tsp of chopped fresh rosemary

- ✓ 2 tbsp of chopped fresh parsley

- ✓ 3 red bell peppers

Procedure:

1. In a large saucepan, add in the quinoa, water, and salt. Stir the ingredients together then set the pan over high heat. Bring the mixture to a boil then adjust the heat to low. Place a lid over the saucepan and simmer for 15 minutes or until all the liquid is absorbed.

2. Remove the lid and wait for 5 minutes before adding in the turkey sausage, chicken stock, olive oil, pecans, parsley,

and rosemary. Stir the ingredients together until well-combined.

3. Cut the red bell peppers in half then remove the membranes and seeds. Boil water and cook the peppers for 5 minutes then drain.

4. Prepare a 13" x 9" baking dish and spray it with cooking spray. Arrange the pepper halves on it. Fill each pepper half with the quinoa mixture then place the baking dish in the oven once done. Bake for 15 minutes at 350F.

Chapter 5: Dessert Recipes

Nutritious Chocolate Pudding

Ingredients:

- ✓ 2 ¼ cups of milk
- ✓ ¼ cup of maple syrup
- ✓ 3 egg yolks
- ✓ ¼ cup of sucanat
- ✓ 3 tbsp of cocoa powder
- ✓ 4 tbsp of arrowroot powder
- ✓ ¼ tsp of salt
- ✓ 2 tsp of vanilla
- ✓ 3 tbsp of butter

Procedure:

1. Prepare a large saucepan and set it over medium heat. Add in the milk, maple syrup, egg yolks, sucanat, cocoa powder, arrowroot powder, and salt. Whisk the ingredients together until properly incorporated.

2. Continue stirring for 7 minutes or until the mixture becomes thick.

3. Take a spoon and dip it into the mixture. If it coats the spoon, remove the pan from the heat immediately.

4. Add in the vanilla and butter then stir to combine.

5. Pour the pudding into ramekins and serve immediately. You can also place it in the refrigerator if you prefer cold chocolate pudding.

No Bake Cookie Bars

Ingredients:

- ✓ 1 cup of natural peanut butter
- ✓ ½ cup of organic coconut oil
- ✓ ½ cup of honey
- ✓ 2 cups of organic dry oats
- ✓ 1 cup of chopped pecans
- ✓ 1 cup of unsweetened coconut flakes, already shredded
- ✓ 1 ¼ cups of dark chocolate chips

Procedure:

1. Prepare a 9" x 13" baking pan and lightly grease it with coconut oil.

2. In a large bowl, add in the dry oats, pecans, coconut flakes, and chocolate chips. Stir the ingredients together until properly combined.

3. Prepare a small saucepan and add in the coconut oil, peanut butter, and honey. Place the pan over low heat and stir the ingredients together. Wait until the coconut oil has mostly melted before removing the pan from the heat.

4. Pour the honey mixture into the bowl with the oats mixture and stir until the ingredients are well-incorporated and the chocolate chips have melted completely.

5. Place the mixture onto the baking pan and spread it evenly.

6. Cover the baking pan with cling wrap and place it inside the refrigerator until the mixture has set.

7. Cut it into bars and serve.

Rustic Bread Pudding

Ingredients:

For the Pudding

- ✓ 2 cups of raw whole milk

- ✓ 2/3 cup of sucanat

- ✓ ¼ cup of pastured butter

- ✓ 3 pastured eggs

- ✓ ¼ tsp of ground nutmeg

- ✓ 2 tsp of cinnamon

- ✓ 1 tsp of vanilla extract

- ✓ ½ cup of raisins

- ✓ 3 cups of sourdough bread, torn into bite-size pieces

For the Sauce

- ✓ 1 cup of half-and-half

- ✓ 1 tsp of vanilla

- ✓ 1/8 cup of sucanat

- ✓ A dash of salt

Procedure:

1. For the sauce: Prepare a saucepan then add in the half-and-half, sucanat, vanilla, and salt. Set the pan over medium heat. Stir for 5 minutes then set it aside until needed.

2. For the pudding: Prepare a saucepan then add in the butter. Wait for the butter to melt completely before adding in the milk. Stir to combine.

3. In a mixing bowl, combine the eggs, sucanat, nutmeg, cinnamon, and vanilla. Whisk the ingredients together until well-combined then gradually add in the milk mixture. Stir the ingredients to combine.

4. Prepare a 1 ½-quart casserole dish and spray it with cooking spray. Place the bread into the dish.

5. Sprinkle the raisins over the bread then pour the mixture on top.

6. Place the casserole dish in the oven and bake for 45 minutes at 350F. Pour the sauce over the pudding once done baking then serve.

Pumpkin Coconut Fudge Squares

Ingredients:

- ✓ 1 can of pumpkin puree
- ✓ 16 dates
- ✓ 2 (200g) packs of coconut butter
- ✓ 1 tsp of cinnamon
- ✓ 1 tsp of vanilla
- ✓ 1 tsp of mixed spice
- ✓ A pinch of sea salt

Procedure:

1. Prepare a bowl of water then add in the dates. Place the bowl in the microwave oven and heat the dates for a couple of minutes until it becomes soft.

2. Place the dates in a food processor and process until it forms a goopy paste.

3. Prepare bowl of hot water and place the coconut butter packs in it. Wait until the coconut butter completely melts before removing the packs from the bowl.

4. In a mixing bowl, add in the pumpkin puree, coconut butter, date paste, cinnamon, mixed spice, vanilla, and sea salt. Stir the ingredients together until it forms a soft ball.

5. Prepare a baking tray and line it with wax paper. Spread the mixture evenly on top of the tray to make ½" thick fudge cake. Sprinkle with extra cinnamon on top then place the tray in the refrigerator until the cake hardens.

6. Cut the fudge cake into squares once set then serve.

Strawberry Gelato

Ingredients:

- ✓ 2 cups of milk
- ✓ 4 egg yolks
- ✓ 1 cup of heavy cream
- ✓ ½ cup of raw honey OR maple syrup
- ✓ ¼ tsp of sea salt
- ✓ 2 cups of fresh strawberries, remove the top part and stems then puree
- ✓ ½ tsp of lemon zest

Procedure:

1. Add in the cream and milk into a saucepan. Stir then bring the mixture to boil. Turn down the heat and simmer for 4 minutes while stirring constantly.

2. In a blender, add in the honey, salt, and egg yolks. Blend until the mixture becomes creamy and smooth.

3. Set the blender on low speed then gradually add in the warm milk into the blender. Perform this step very slowly to prevent the hot milk from cooking the eggs.

4. Return the mixture into the saucepan and adjust the heat to medium-low. Cook for 10 minutes while stirring constantly or until the mixture begins to thicken.

5. Add in the lemon zest and strawberry puree into the pan. Stir the ingredients to combine.

6. Place the mixture in the refrigerator for 4 hours or until the mixture has cooled completely. Once cool, freeze the mixture for 2 hours then add it into the blender to process until it becomes smooth. Replace the mixture into the freezer and wait for another 3 hours or until the mixture hardens. Serve and enjoy.

Conclusion

Thank you again for purchasing this book!

I hope this book was able to help you to start a healthier lifestyle beginning with your diet.

The next step is to apply and incorporate these recipes into your diet plan so you can gradually adjust your appetite to this diet.

Finally, if you enjoyed this book, please take the time to share your thoughts and post a positive review on Amazon. It'd be greatly appreciated!

In addition, please remember to check out our Facebook page in order to find other resources and upcoming promotions:

https://www.facebook.com/joypublishing

With sincere thanks,

Emma Rose

Preview Of "Paleo Free Diet Guide for Beginners: Over 50 Paleo Diet Recipes for Fast Weight Loss and Optimal Health"

Introduction

I want to thank you and congratulate you for purchasing the book, *"Paleo Free Diet Guide for Beginners: Over 50 Paleo Diet Recipes for Optimal Health and Fast Weight Loss"*.

This book contains everything you might need to know when it comes to getting started with the Paleo diet. It is provided in an easily digestible format that allows you to better absorb the information. There are no complicated explanations about how it works! You'll be given what you need straight up so you won't have to waste time trying to understand exactly what the diet is. Whether it's for your overall good health or to lose a few pounds, Paleo can certainly help you with it. To help you get started, we'll do the same and start you off with 50 of the best Paleo recipes that you can slowly but surely shift your everyday menu to.

It's never easy changing a diet. I often fall into self pity when I can no longer have the foods I enjoy. Either I feel sorry for myself or I get rebellious and binge and anything and everything. I always knew the value of eating healthy. I could just never bring myself to do it. It wasn't until I had a miscarriage that I got serious about my health. I have made drastic changes that others just don't understand. But the pay off is the weight I've lost and the better health I'm experiencing.

My hope for you is not to be on another "diet." This isn't a restriction diet like Atkins. The goal is to have a lifestyle change. Lifestyle changes are more sustainable and maintain weight loss long term compared to restriction diets. The change is hard to start but worth it when you commit. The trick is to get the momentum to start.

Thanks again for purchasing this book. I hope you enjoy reading it and eating the recipes from it!

With gratitude,

Emma   Rose

Chapter 1 – What Is the Paleo Diet?

The Paleo Diet is known by many names such as the cavemen diet, stone age diet and hunter-gatherer diet, to name a few. The concept behind this diet follows that of the Paleolithic era before the development of agriculture. Essentially, you consume the same foods that the cavemen used to eat. The focus is on eating food closest to its natural, unprocessed state. The cavemen would gather their food from any source available whether it was wild animals, berries, vegetables, or fruits. As a result, they were strong, fit, and healthy for thousand of years.

This type of diet is still very young, less than fifty years only, but more in depth researches and studies are being conducted to increase the information and knowledge on this diet. The results of previous studies conducted on the Paleo diet reveal the improvement of health to the people involved. This is attributed to the fact that no processed foods and additives are included. The Paleo Diet is a diet that works with our genetics – before machinery and processing got involved. Foods that were not available during the Paleolithic time such as dairy products, salt, sugar and grains are not included in the preparation of the Paleo diet.

The modern diet predominately consumed in the Western world is full of refined foods, trans fats, salt and sugar. These ingredients are known to indirectly cause diseases such as hypertension, diabetes, strokes, obesity and other heart problems. The list goes on even further with the increase diagnosis of cancer, Parkinson's, Alzheimer's, depression and infertility. "What an extraordinary achievement for a civilization: to have developed the one diet that reliably makes its people sick!" (Michael Pollen, Food Rules: An Eater's Manual, Penguin Books 2009).

Foods included in the Paleo Diet

- Fruit

- Vegetables

- Lean Meat

- Seafood

- Nuts/Seeds

- Healthy Fats (eg. coconut, avocado, nuts and seeds, olive oil, grass fed butter)

Foods NOT included in the Paleo Diet

- Dairy

- Grain

- Processed Food

Why not grain?

You may be surprised to see that grains are not included in the Paleo Diet. We are accustomed to grains being a part of a balanced diet. However, our bodies are not designed to deal with the nutritional components of grains such as gluten, lectin, and phytates.

Gluten is a protein substance found in wheat, barley and rye. Many people are discovering that their bodies are gluten sensitive and are eliminating gluten from their diet. The most extreme case of gluten sensitivity is Celiac Disease. Individuals with this disease can pick up the minutest trace of gluten and react immediately.

Lectin binds to insulin receptors and can also cause leptin resistance.

Phytates cause minerals to become unavailable during digestion.

Why is dairy a problem?

When purchasing milk, you need to be mindful of the source.

Check out the rest of "Paleo Free Diet Guide for Beginners: Over 50 Paleo Diet Recipes for Fast Weight Loss and Optimal Health" on Amazon

Or go to: http://amzn.to/1jIJUFX

Detox Diet Guide

Lose Weight Quickly, Achieve Optimal Health and Feel Energized Through the 10 Day Detox

Emma Rose

Table of Contents

Introduction

I want to thank you and congratulate you for purchasing the book, *"Detox Diet Guide: Lose Weight Quickly, Achieve Optimal Health and Feel Energized Through the 10 Day Detox"*.

This book contains proven steps and strategies on how to not just simply flush out toxic substances from our bodies, but to also enhance the way our bodies naturally flush out those toxins.

It also contains other important information such as the most common toxins that are found in the environment that we unknowingly consume, the many ways our bodies naturally detoxify themselves, the things one must and must not do within the ten days of the detox diet, detoxification recipes that can be easily prepared, and some important reminders that must be taken before, during, and after the detox diet.

Thanks again for purchasing this book. I hope you enjoy it! Please take some time to stop by and LIKE our Facebook page:

https://www.facebook.com/joypublishing

With gratitude,

Emma Rose

Chapter 1: Toxins and the Body

As the human body does its usual processes, some things need to be expelled. These are usually waste products made as a result of filtering out substances not needed by the body. There is a reason for the so-called "calls of nature" – which are peeing and releasing excrement.

But sometimes, those unwanted substances can build up in the organs and the bodily systems that comprise them. If there are too much of those substances, they will cause all sorts of harm to the overall bodily functions that can lead to various ailments.

The Top 10 List of Most Common Toxins

Human civilization evolves as a result of the desire of the people to live more comfortably and conveniently. But in the process of that evolution, it has unknowingly unleashed a cavalcade of impurities that do not just pollute the environment, but also the human body. Despite the many efforts by several government agencies and private individuals to thwart the sources of those impurities, there are traces of those impurities that still linger around. Those traces remain in the air, in the soil, in several bodies of water – and eventually, in the foods that humanity consumes.

According to Dr. Joseph Mercola, a well-known personality in the US wellness movement and owner and founder of Mercola.com (one of the most-trusted health websites), the ten most common toxic substances that are still prevalent in the environment to this day are the following:

1. Polychlorinated biphenyls, or PCBs, were commonly dumped by factories into nearby bodies of water. Due to their toxicity, PCBs were banned decades ago. However, traces of PCBs can still be found in those bodies of water since the toxic substances do not break down easily even after all those years. Fish that swim in those bodies of water still consume PCBs

unknowingly. As people still eat those fish, they will also ingest PCBs that will contribute to ailments such as cancer and brain defects in newborn babies.

2. Pesticides, while they do kill pests as their name says, are the major contributors of cancer. As farms still use synthetic pesticides such as weed killers, fungi killers, and insect killers; residues of those pesticides still remain in as much as 50 to 90 percent of US farm produce. Furthermore, there are bug sprays used to kill cockroaches and other unwanted insects in homes. Those bug sprays also contain the same carcinogenic substances as farm-focused pesticides. Besides cancer, pesticides also cause Parkinson's disease, miscarriage, nerve damage, birth defects, and getting in the way of nutrient absorption.

3. Fungal toxins not just come in the form of poisonous mushrooms. The most common of those fungal toxins is mould. Mould thrives in moist places such as bathrooms and kitchens; and can even sustain in vulnerable foods such as peanuts, wheat, and corn. One in three people are allergic to this fungal toxin. If left unchecked, mould causes cancer, heart disease, asthma, multiple sclerosis, and diabetes.

4. Phthalates are commonly found in plastic products and are responsible for softening them, making them easier to mold. They can seep into foodstuffs and drinks that are placed inside plastic food containers and plastic bottles. The result of ingesting too much phthalates is hormonal imbalance, since the substances resemble naturally-produced hormones. In children, phthalates can stunt their growth.

5. Volatile organic compounds, or VOCs, are commonly found in several household products such as air fresheners, cleaning fluids, mothballs, and varnishes. VOCs aid in air pollution and cause several sicknesses such as cancer, irritation of eyes and lungs, headaches, dizziness, and impaired memory.

6. Dioxins are some of the pollutants that are produced when something is burned, especially in massive quantities. As they

are released into the air, humans not just breathe in the dioxins. Livestock can also inhale those toxins and settle in their fats even after they are brought to the slaughterhouse to be made into meat. Dioxins cause cancer, stunted growth, reproductive system impairments, skin disorders such as acne, and slight damage to the liver.

7. Asbestos was a popular insulation material, but it was banned in the seventies due to its carcinogenic effects. Traces of asbestos can still be found in old homes that did not have their insulations replaced. Besides cancer, asbestos causes scarring on the lung tissue.

8. Toxic heavy metals such as lead, arsenic, and mercury can still be found in various objects such as cheaply-made toys, preserved wood, antiperspirants, and building materials. Once those metals are inhaled or ingested, they can cause cancer, brain and nerve disorders such as Alzheimer's disease, nausea, lesser amounts of red and white blood cells, and abnormal heartbeats.

9. Chloroform is a common chemical that is used to make other chemicals. It is prevalent in the air, in water, and in food. It can cause cancer, infertility, birth defects, headaches, dizziness, and damage to the liver and kidneys.

10. Chlorine is commonly found in water as it is used to purify it. Whether from the typical drinking water or from a swimming pool, too much of chlorine will cause all sorts of respiratory problems such as sore throat, accumulation of fluid in the lungs, and asthma.

Based on this list, many of those toxins in the environment are brought about by humanity's modern lifestyles. Before they do undue harm to the body, especially the dreaded cancer, they must be flushed out promptly.

Other Sources of Toxins

Besides the ten most common toxic substances, there are also other toxins that can be found in almost everything in the modern world. It is inevitable that one must intake those toxins unknowingly, one way or the other.

The two most popular vices, which are smoking and drinking, are the other major reasons for the body's toxicity. Both alcohol and nicotine have been proven many times by the scientific community to be not just toxic, but also addicting. Those two substances also alter the brain's functions. Other toxic substances include caffeine, empty sugars, and saturated fats. The latter two are especially notorious for being fat fodder since they cannot be processed into needed energy.

Many cosmetics today also contain toxic substances such as VOCs that can be absorbed into the skin. Some cosmetics producers have already taken steps in ridding their beauty products of those toxins.

Taking too many medications all at once can also cause the body to be laced with toxins, since they are not properly eliminated from the body. If the body feels too taxed from a cornucopia of meds, a consultation with the doctor will help.

There are also naturally-occurring toxins that are used by certain plants and animals as defense mechanisms against invaders. Snakes and jellyfish have highly deadly toxins and should not be consumed as food. A Japanese dish called *fugu* uses a type of blowfish that releases toxins which will certainly kill someone who eats an improperly-prepared version of the dish.

Processed foods, especially canned goods, are also a major source of toxins. While those foods contain preservatives that prolong their shelf lives, they unknowingly unleash a world of hurt on one who voraciously eats these. Needless to say, one must balance those foods out with naturally-grown foods.

Chapter 2: Why Must We Detoxify?

Detoxification is not just the simple flushing out of unwanted substances when the body cannot handle expelling them on its own. It is also the purging of impure thoughts in the mind that cause all sorts of decisions to inhale and ingest several toxins, whether knowingly or unknowingly, into the body. To ensure that an individual is rightfully clean in both body and mind, all sorts of unwanted things must be eliminated, especially in the detox diet.

The Body Does It Own Job...

The excretory system does its job of purging waste substances from the body via its two major processes: urination and release of excrement. Urination is obviously handled by the urinary system, while the release of excrement is handled by the lower parts of the digestive system.

The urinary system's main actor is the kidneys. The kidneys filter unwanted stuff such as ammonia, urea, uric acid, and excess salt and water from the blood as well as other bodily fluids. Those unwanted stuff then get to the bladder, which acts as a temporary storage. If the bladder gets full, the stuff gets expelled out of the urethra in the form of urine. Ammonia is a byproduct of the breakdown and usage of protein for the body's energy, while urea and uric acid are less toxic substances that result from the breakdown of ammonia.

The lower parts of the digestive system consist of the liver, the intestines, and the colon. The liver does its job of breaking down foreign substances so that the kidneys can have an easier job filtering them out as urine. The intestines and the colon facilitate the expelling of solid waste substances in the form of feces. The colon, in particular, absorbs trace minerals such as potassium and sends them to the bloodstream before they are included as feces that will be expelled by pooping.

Another natural detoxifier found in the human body is the lymphatic system. The lymphatic system contains lymph nodes that are scattered throughout the body but are interconnected. Those nodes provide the body with immunity, complementing the immune system, by filtering out unwelcome invaders such as bacteria, viruses, old red blood cells, and other toxic substances.

Other parts of the excretory system consist of the lungs and skin. The lungs expel excess water and carbon dioxide when someone breathes out. The skin kicks out excess water, salt, uric acid, and excess trace minerals in the form of sweat.

...But It Is Not Enough in the Modern Age

However, as demonstrated in the previous chapter, there are far too many substances that are deemed toxic in the wrong amounts. With humanity's modern lifestyles, the body does not know what to make of the increasing number of unwelcome invaders in its insides. These usually never get flushed out as urine and feces, but instead accumulate in the body fat.

As the invaders multiply and never get flushed out, they get in the way of the body's usual processes and will cause several problems such as depleted energy levels, unnatural weight gain, and various diseases that target the major body systems.

Another thing that is not helping the body in its natural detoxification process is the busy and hectic schedules people normally have. Because those people have no time to perform even mundane healthy tasks such as drinking adequate water, the body never gets its supply of natural detox assistants. Couple the lack of those assistants with stress and it will be a recipe for disaster.

Therefore, it is important that in this world of toxicity, people must amplify their bodily defenses against all sorts of foreign toxic substances by enhancing the many components of the excretory system such as the kidneys, the liver, the intestines, and the colon. With the contaminants out of the way, the body's natural healing processes also get their groove back. As the major organ systems work hand-in-hand, the benefits that are felt in one particular system will spread towards the other systems.

In short, steeling the body and its functions, especially the excretory functions, is one of the first lines of defense against toxin-induced sicknesses. There will be a marked loss in weight, since the excessive fats as well as the toxins they contain are properly expelled. There will also be renewed liveliness since the bodily functions that have something to do with the intake and processing of energy sources are no longer clogged by invasive toxins.

Why the Mind Is Also Important in Detoxification

The decisions a person makes, no matter how small they are, can contribute to huge consequences. For example, if one decides to commute to a bar, he or she gets all sorts of toxins in the process – airborne impurities from urban roads, food additives from the snacks he or she eats while commuting, nicotine and other chemicals from tobacco smoke generated by smokers inside and outside the bar, and alcohol from the hard drinks he or she consumes while in the bar.

Therefore, it is important that a person must think thoroughly and deeply before settling on a decision that will make him or her take in all those unwanted toxins along the way. Yes, this may turn him or her into a control freak, but there are also decisions that will endow him or her with long-term benefits. Remember, detoxification starts in the mind. The decisions that lead to the unknowing intake of toxins must be sorted out and eliminated from the usual routines first.

Chapter 3: The Crucial Ten Days

There are several forms of detoxification, and they more often than not involve ingesting special liquids and solids, cleansing the colon, foot baths and foot pads, spas and saunas, and fasting. But they also cost money, are always focused on the short-term effects, and may not deliver the detoxification results one desires. The best form of the detox diet must involve getting rid of major sources of toxins, ingesting more of the substances that will greatly assist the body's natural detoxification processes, never integrating any form of starvation or elimination of a major food group from the diet, and clearing the mind of impure thoughts that lead to impure actions. This way, the diet will grant long-term effects of well-being. As a beneficial consequence, this diet will cost little to no money, except for the money to be spent on detoxifying foods and drinks.

The ten days this detox diet contains are important to ensure natural weight loss and general well-being. And even after the diet period ends, some good habits contained in this diet, particularly the continued eating of healthy foods, must still be kept. This is to ensure that the person undergoing this diet will transition into a healthy lifestyle.

Preparing for the Diet

One important thing to do when undergoing this diet, or any other diet for that matter, is to not rush in immediately. A crash diet will have nasty consequences such as abrupt changing of body patterns that lead to all sorts of ailments as well as retention of the weight one lost during the diet routine. Therefore, one must start slow and transition into the diet carefully.

Not rushing in also applies to the chewing of food. The body needs some time to digest the food. Never treat the ten days of the diet like some kind of work deadline.

The usual vice-based sources of toxins, which are tobacco and alcohol, must be eliminated first. While dealing with the withdrawal effects of both of those substances may be difficult, timely help from a doctor who has a specialization in several types of addictions and substance abuse will lessen the difficulty.

In the three days before the actual start of the diet, rid the pantry and fridge of tempting foodstuffs that are loaded with empty calories. These include sweets and most forms of processed foods and fast food. At the same time, steadily increase the intake of fruits and vegetables – *especially organic ones*. As much as possible, turn the veggies into freshly-prepared salads and/or lightly steam them. As for the fruits, eat them raw and/or turn them into natural juices.

Since pesticide residue in fruits and vegetables is inevitable, the use of fruit and vegetable washes must be prioritized.

The intake of caffeine must be slowly and surely reduced to prevent withdrawal symptoms such as headaches. Switching to decaf coffee and low-caffeine teas such as green tea will help, as is the trick of diluting regular coffee and tea in huge amounts of water.

And speaking of water, the time-tested advice of eight to ten glasses of water a day will especially help the detox diet become successful. Drink it throughout the ten days of the diet.

Aromatherapy using essential oils is helpful, as this therapy helps to calm the mind in order for it to prepare for the rigors of the critical ten days.

Finally, before embarking on the detox diet itself, please consult a registered dietician who can recommend the detoxifying foods to be eaten based on your genetic makeup. Furthermore, *do not stop* taking prescribed medicine, as discontinuing medications can have devastating effects on the body. Diets are not meant to be one-man shows, especially if the individual still has to learn much about the intricacies of diet programs like this.

Eat and Drink Them

With the transition phase over, it is time to actually start the detox diet. Here is a comprehensive list of foods and drinks that must be ingested during the ten crucial days of the diet.

1. Organic fruits and vegetables are the main focus of the detox diet. It does not matter what the size or type of fruit or vegetable one will be consuming – as long as it is free of pesticides and synthetic fertilizers and is grown using age-old farming techniques, it certainly counts. Eat a good variety of fruits and vegetables to round out all the necessary nutrients.

2. Brown rice is much healthier compared to the typical white rice. As white rice is a result of the milling process, brown rice retains some nutrients that are usually lost during milling. This type of rice is also a rich source of fiber, which will aid in flushing the toxins out via the intestines and the colon.

3. Herbs are permissible, since they are also plants. Use them to flavor the dishes as well as utilize them for aromatherapy. Herbal teas are also a-OK, since they do not contain caffeine at all. As with fruits and vegetables, herbs must not have traces of anything toxic.

4. Whole-grain products, much like brown rice, do not undergo the nutrient-losing milling process. They are also rich sources of fiber. Whole-grain products include whole wheat bread, bran, and rolled oats.

5. Seaweeds such as kelp and *nori* wrappers used for sushi are also plant-based. They can also be consumed the same way as typical veggies do.

6. Beans such as green peas, chick peas, lentils, kidney beans, and black beans are permitted.

7. One can go nuts with nuts and seeds. Allowable things include almonds, cashews, walnuts, watermelon seeds, pumpkin

seeds, sunflower seeds, and sesame seeds. As a general rule, pick only raw, unsalted nuts and seeds.

8. Coconuts, while they are not actually nuts, are also allowed. There are several coconut-based consumables such as coconut water and coconut oil. One can also eat fresh coconut meat straight from the source.

9. Plant-based oils are encouraged. Olive oil, especially the extra virgin kind, is highly recommended.

10. Round out the protein-based nutrition with plant-based protein sources such as soy. Soy milk and tofu are easily-acquired sources of plant-based protein.

11. All sorts of edible mushrooms are permitted. Portobello and shiitake mushrooms can act as good substitutes for meat.

12. Natural sweeteners such as raw honey and natural maple syrup are permitted.

13. Besides herbs, other natural condiments that are tolerable include apple cider vinegar, sea salt, and mustard.

14. If there is still a desire to eat meat and get adequate protein, go with lean meats such as fish and organic chicken. Eggs are also on the list, as long as they are organic.

Never Eat and Drink Them

Meanwhile, these are the foods and drinks to avoid during the detox diet phase.

1. In general, non-lean types of red meat are off-limits. Canned meat is especially forbidden.

2. All forms of processed foods containing all sorts of additives and preservatives are out of the question. On a related note, artificial sweeteners and processed condiments are also out.

3. Typical white sugar and brown sugar are verboten, as well as high-fructose syrups.

4. Corn must be avoided as it is acid-forming. The acid in question is uric acid. Furthermore, the corn kernels that are indigestible will make bathroom breaks more excruciating.

5. While nuts are OK, peanuts and peanut butter are usually excluded.

6. Milk is normally not allowed, but half a cup of yogurt containing good bacteria per day is an exception to that.

7. Caffeine is another typical forbidden substance.

8. Shortening and margarine are inadmissible.

9. While fish is OK, other seafoods are not.

Other Cleansing Procedures

There are many variations of the detox diet, but the one being presented in this book will not involve complicated doohickeys and specialized food and drinks to amplify the detoxification effect. Here are some things one can also do during the ten days of the diet.

With all the conveniences of Internet-based connectivity, sometimes too much is too much. Dedicate one of the ten days, or even all ten days, to a temporary break from technology. Put away the smartphone or tablet, avoid touching the computer, and never be tempted to go online just about anywhere. Take the time off from technology to visit someplace serene, like a retreat house. This technology break will clear the mind of all sorts of burdening thoughts that may poison one's thinking the same way that bodily toxins do.

Take some time off to scrape the tongue. Tongue scraping is a practice in ayurvedic medicine, or ancient Hindu medicine, where all the impurities built up on the tongue are removed. Tongue scrapers can be bought for cheap at drug store.

Try to write all the stored thoughts and feelings, even negative ones, into a diary or notebook. Releasing all the stored strong emotions to a diary or notebook has a cathartic effect, since keeping those emotions locked away will eventually take the toll on one's health.

Another mind-cleansing procedure one can do during the ten days is meditation. Meditation also helps clear the mind of toxic thoughts that lead to stress, which then slows down the liver's detoxification process. Yoga is especially helpful as a meditation tool. You may also augment your meditation by doing deep breathing exercises or visualizing relaxing images such as watching the sunset at the beach.

Get enough dosages of vitamin C. While the vitamin is better known for boosting immunity, it also helps the body with the production of glutathione. Glutathione may be better known as a skin rejuvenating agent, but it also exists in the liver as a detoxification aid. Citrus fruits are the best-known sources of vitamin C.

Enhance blood circulation, since poor blood circulation will hamper the flushing out of impurities from the blood. Exercise is a guaranteed way to get that blood pumping.

Keep in mind that not all bacteria are bad. Good bacteria mostly reside in the intestines, aiding in digestion and preventing bad bacteria from releasing toxins that can be deployed in the bloodstream. Help the good bacteria by taking probiotic drinks.

Chapter 4: Detoxification Recipes

Breakfast Recipes

Gut-Busting Oatmeal Bowl

Ingredients:

- 1-2 cups oatmeal

- 1-2 cups water or nut milk

- A mixture of fresh berries and fresh fruits, all sliced

Procedure:

1. Prepare the oatmeal as indicated in the packaging.

2. While hot, pour the berries and fruits onto the prepared oatmeal, and mix.

Berry Blast Smoothie

Ingredients:

- 1-2 cups mixed fresh berries
- 1-2 cups protein powder
- 1-2 cups ice cubes

Procedure:

1. Throw all the ingredients into a blender, and hit puree.
2. Serve the smoothie in a tall glass.

Lunch Recipes

Veggie Cavalcade Salad with Tofu

Ingredients:

- 6-8 pieces of any whole vegetable (for greens, an amount of at least five leaves equals one whole piece)

- 1-2 pieces tofu, diced

- 4-5 teaspoons extra virgin olive oil

- 2 teaspoons fresh lemon juice

- 1 teaspoon freshly-chopped herbs of choice

Procedure:

1. Fry the tofu in 2-3 teaspoons olive oil until slightly browned. Set aside.

2. Slice and/or dice the vegetables into reasonably-sized pieces. Leave the greens untouched.

3. Pour all the vegetables and the tofu into a bowl. Mix completely.

4. Combine 2 teaspoons olive oil, the lemon juice, and the herbs to make the dressing.

5. Pour the dressing all over the salad. Mix completely.

Special Omelet Rice

Ingredients:

- 3-5 organic eggs

- Fresh or dried herbs (any variety), to taste

- 2-3 teaspoons extra virgin olive oil

- 1-2 cups cooked brown rice

Procedure:

1. Beat the eggs into a scramble while adding the herbs.

2. Pour the olive oil into a heated pan. Wait until the oil is hot.

3. Pour the egg and herb mixture until the omelet is formed. Turn over to ensure proper cooking.

4. Once the omelet is out of the pan, place the brown rice inside it. Make sure the omelet wraps around the rice.

5. Serve hot with mustard.

Dinner Recipes

The Steamed Medley

Ingredients:

- 1 slice salmon

- 5-10 pieces broccoli and asparagus (can be of any combination)

- 1/4 cup fresh lemon juice

- Fresh or dried herbs (any variety), to taste

Procedure:

1. In a steamer or a rice cooker with a steaming basket, arrange the salmon slice and the broccoli and asparagus pieces so that the steam will be evenly distributed.

2. Sprinkle the salmon and the vegetables with the lemon juice and fresh herbs.

3. Begin steaming the salmon and the vegetables. Seven to ten minutes is enough for the lemon and the herbs to seep into the steamed content.

4. Serve hot.

Glorified Bunch of Small Potatoes

Ingredients:

- 6 ounces small potatoes

- 4 tablespoons extra virgin olive oil

- Any natural condiment of choice

Procedure:

1. Gently simmer the potatoes in water for 5-10 minutes. Drain them off afterwards. Retain the peels beforehand.

2. Heat the olive oil in a roasting tin, but not to burning levels.

3. Roast every side of the potatoes until crisp and golden brown. This will take at most 45 minutes.

4. Serve hot with the condiment of choice.

Snack and Drink Recipes

Veggie Brown Rice Sushi

Ingredients:

- 1 cup cooked brown rice
- 1 *nori* wrapper
- Any sliced or diced vegetable that can fit inside the sushi

Procedure:

1. Mold the brown rice into any shape, whether in a tube form or rolled into a ball. The important thing is that the vegetable must fit inside the sushi.

2. Wrap the *nori* wrapper around the formed brown rice.

3. Repeat steps 1 and 2 for any remaining amounts of vegetables, brown rice, and the *nori* wrapper.

Stretched Herbal Iced Tea

Ingredients:

- 1 bag herbal tea (any kind)
- 1 citrus fruit of choice (e.g. lemon or orange)
- 1 cup briskly-boiled water
- 2-3 cups lukewarm water
- Several ice cubes
- Honey, to taste

Procedure:

1. Depending on the strength of the resultant tea, submerge one teabag into briskly-boiled water.

2. Meanwhile, cut the citrus fruit of choice into slices that can be fit inside a glass.

3. Place the fruit slices into a tall glass that can accommodate at least five cups.

4. Carefully pour both the brewed tea and the lukewarm water into the tall glass at a distance of at least 12 inches from the glass. This is where the "stretched" part comes from, and one must avoid spills during the stretching process.

5. Add some dollops of honey based on the preferred amount of sweetness.

6. Finally, add the ice cubes.

Fruity Shaved Ice

Ingredients:

- 1-2 cups shaved ice
- 1/2-1 cup natural unsweetened fruit juice of any kind

Procedure:

1. Place the shaved ice in either a wide glass or a bowl.
2. Pour the unsweetened fruit juice on top of the shaved ice, and enjoy.

Note: One can replace shaved ice with shaved or crushed frozen fruit.

Chapter 5: Some Friendly Reminders

As with every other diet program on the planet, care, precise planning, patience, and perseverance must be taken to heart when undergoing the detoxification diet. Even in a short period like ten days, many things will happen. To ensure that the detox diet will become a success that will beget many more successes in the realm of the healthy lifestyle, keep the following friendly reminders in mind.

Do Not Starve

Other detox diets recommend taking only the formulas they sell themselves. Indeed, they may contain needed plant-based nourishment needed for detoxification, but the makers of those diets often forget that an imbalanced diet that is lacking in calories will prove detrimental to the body. Not only will the energy levels be depleted, but the metabolism process will also be slowed down. One unpleasant aftereffect is the tendency to eat more, especially unhealthy foods, once the diet period is over. This will make natural weight loss almost unachievable. Even worse, the lack of micronutrients in these other detox diets will lead to malnutrition that is based on micronutrient deficiency, which opens yet another floodgate of diseases. Other nasty effects of other detox crash diets include muscle degeneration, since the muscles have no source of energy to turn to, and an imbalance in blood sugar levels.

Hence, this detox diet espouses the idea that *forced starvation is absolutely prohibited.* Just eat the recommended foods at will and in good, moderated amounts.

Expect to Pee (and Poop and Sweat) a Lot

Since the detox diet enhances the body's natural detox functions, expect one undergoing the diet to pee a lot. Water, in particular, helps in flushing out toxins.

Excessive peeing not just happens when the detox diet goes overboard. Excessive sweating also happens, as well as the resultant excrement being too liquid and nasty-smelling. Peeing, pooping, and sweating too much can lead to dehydration if the amount of fluids being taken is not immediately replenished.

Dehydration is not just the depletion of the body's water, but is also the disrupted balance of fluids and electrolytes that can lead to ailments such as gastrointestinal distress, headaches, fatigue, irritability, skin irritations, circulatory problems, kidney failure, and heat stroke. Death also awaits one who is severely dehydrated.

To counteract dehydration, do not depend on fluids and fluids alone, unlike what some detox diets emphasize. Be well-balanced in both solids and liquids to avoid lost hours as a result of abnormally frequent trips to the bathroom.

Want a Colonic? No Thanks

Another form of the detox therapy involves cleansing the colon and intestines of toxins that may be released into the bloodstream. However, as demonstrated in the third chapter, there are beneficial bacteria that reside in the colon and intestines. If those bacteria are flushed out, the normal digestive process will be hampered, and the bad bacteria will have a good time releasing more toxins since their rivals are gone. The flushing out of good bacteria also results from the detox diet going beyond the recommended ten days.

Another bad effect of colon cleansing is dehydration, for the same reasons demonstrated in the previous section. Trace minerals such as potassium are also lost during the cleansing process, which contributes to dehydration. Other side effects of colon cleansing include nausea and vomiting.

Diet as an End to the Means, Not a Means to the End

People who want the figures of their dreams often forget that dieting is not really meant to immediately shed unwanted pounds. Dieting is truly meant for improved nourishment and nutrition. The notions of shedding that slab or beer belly in preparation for an event like showing off in a bikini should be disposed of. A proper mindset must be established first when doing the detox diet or any other diet for that matter.

As stated before, the detox diet being demonstrated in this book should be a transitional phase to a healthier lifestyle. Thinking in the long term when dieting is certainly better than thinking in the short term. One should remember that dieting must be an end to unhealthy habits and not a means to end that "awful" figure.

Conclusion

Thank you again for purchasing *"Detox Diet Guide: Lose Weight Quickly, Achieve Optimal Health and Feel Energized Through the 10 Day Detox"*!

I hope this book was able to help you to understand the ins and outs of the detox diet and why it is important to achieve a major change in only a short time.

Are you ready for the change? Tony Robbins says in order to create effective change, you need to start by being disgusted with where you are at. Are you disgusted with your health or body? Is it an ABSOLUTE MUST to change...not another moment? You need to feel the pain of where you are at to get the urgency to change and manifest the momentum to take action.

The next step is to consult your doctor or dietician before embarking on such a diet. And once you are given the final OK, you can then consult various more detoxification recipes based on the comprehensive list of allowable foods and drinks in this book. The recipes given in this book is just a starting point.

Finally, if you enjoyed this book, please take the time to share your thoughts and post a review on Amazon. It would be greatly appreciated!

I would love for you to share your experiences, stories and encouragements with me. My email address is

emmarosekindle@gmail.com

In addition, please remember to check out our Facebook page in order to find other resources and upcoming promotions:

https://www.facebook.com/joypublishing

With sincere thanks,

Emma Rose

Preview of "Raw Food Diet Guide: Lose Weight Quickly, Achieve Optimal Health and Feel Energized with the Raw Food Diet and Raw Food Recipes"

Chapter 1

An Overview of the Raw Food Diet

The concept of the raw food diet is simple – cooking diminishes the nutritional value of food. Even though most of the food items in the diet are consumed while it is raw, heating is acceptable provided that the temperature stays between the range of 104 to 118°F or below.

Since cooking is perceived to kill off enzymes naturally found in food, raw food practitioners choose to avoid cooked food. As a matter of fact, overconsumption of cooked food forces the body to work overtime in order to produce more enzymes to support normal bodily functions. In the long run, the lack of enzymes can instigate a lot of problems involving a person's health, particularly accelerated aging, nutrient deficiency, weight gain and digestive problems.

Going raw can prove to be challenging, especially for those that are just starting out. It takes a lot of discipline to stick to the principles of the diet. Moreover, extra effort is required mentally and physically. When it comes to preparing your daily raw meals, your options are limited. Here are some of the procedures you may apply when organizing your meal plan:

- *Germination* – this is the process of soaking in water for a certain period of time. The recommended amount of time differs from one person to another but for raw foodists, the safest bet is to soak overnight.

- *Sprouting* – this comes after germination. After the beans, legumes or seeds are soaked, they may then be sprouted. Items should be left at room temperature until a sprout comes out of it. These sprouts may then be used for preparing food but should be rinsed and drained thoroughly beforehand.

- *Blending* – involves the use of a blender or food processor in order to create sauces, smoothies, or soup among others.

- *Dehydrating* – employs an equipment known as a dehydrator, which simulates sun drying. Common products of dehydrators are crackers, croutons, raisins, fruit leathers, sundried tomatoes, breads and kale chips.

- *Pickling* – a method of preserving food by marinating in a brine.

- *Juicing* – the process of extracting of vitamins, minerals and natural juices from plant tissues, particularly raw fruits and vegetables.

- *Fermentation* – process of converting sugar to carbon dioxide through the use of yeast.

Now that you know what procedures are available to you when preparing your raw meals, the next thing to know is which particular equipment/s you need to use. Below are some of the staple equipment that can be seen in every raw foodist's kitchen:

- *Dehydrator*—it is an enclosed container that has heating elements that can warm at low temperatures. It has a fan that blows warm air onto the food.

- *Spiral Slicer* — slices vegetables into spiral shapes

- *Thermometer* — to ensure that temperature stays below 118°F when heating food.

- *Trays* — for soaking and sprouting beans, legumes or seeds

- *Sprouters* or *mason jars*

- *Food processor*

- *Blender*

- *Juicer*

Check out the rest of "Raw Food Diet Guide: Lose Weight Quickly, Achieve Optimal Health and Feel Energized with the Raw Food Diet and Raw Food Recipes" on Amazon

Or go to: http://amzn.to/1xt93sY

Check Out My Other Books

Below you'll find some of my other books also available on Amazon and Kindle. Search for these titles on the Amazon website to find them.

Paleo Free Diet Guide for Beginners: Over 50 Paleo Free Recipes for Optimal Health & Fast Weight Loss

Paleo Desserts: Satisfy Your Sweet Tooth With Over 100 Quick & Easy Paleo Dessert Recipes & Paleo Baking Recipes

Raw Food Diet Guide: Lose Weight Quickly, Achieve Optimal Health & Feel Energized with the Raw Food Diet & Raw Food Recipes

Clean Eating Guide: Lose Weight Quickly, Achieve Optimal Health & Feel Energized with Clean Eating For Busy Families & Clean Eating Recipes

Alkaline Diet Guide: Lose Weight Quickly, Achieve Optimal Health & Feel Energized with the Alkaline Diet & Alkaline Recipes

Coconut Flour Recipes for Optimal Health & Quick Weight Loss: Gluten Free Recipes for Celiac Disease, Gluten Sensitivities & Paleo Free Diets

Almond Flour Recipes for Optimal Health & Quick Weight Loss: Gluten Free Recipes for Celiac Disease, Gluten Sensitivities & Paleo Free Diets

Wheat Free Diet for Beginners: Lose Weight Quickly, Achieve Optimal Health & Feel Energized with Gluten Free Recipes for Celiac Disease, Gluten Sensitivities & Paleo Free Diets

Detox Diet Guide: Lose Weight Quickly, Achieve Optimal Health & Feel Energized Through the 10 Day Detox

Sugar Detox Guide for Beginners: Lose Weight Quickly, Achieve Optimal Health, Feel Energized & Eliminate Sugar Cravings Naturally

Ketogenic Diet Guide for Beginners: How to Achieve Rapid Weight Loss, Optimal Health & Unstoppable Energy with Ketogenic Diet Recipes

Anti Inflammatory Diet for Beginners: Lose Weight Fast, Optimize Health, Slow Aging, Fight Inflammation, Conquer Pain & Increase Energy with the Anti Inflammation Diet Recipes

One Last Thing...

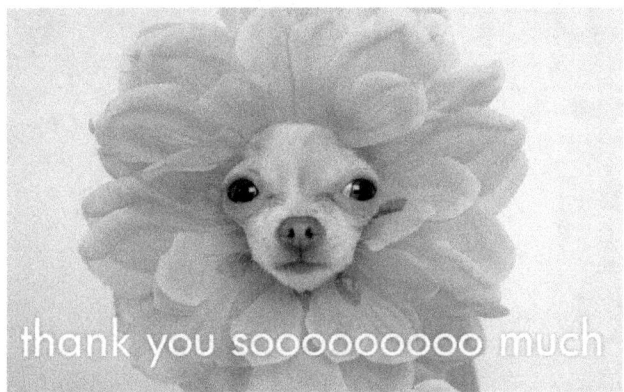

thank you soooooooooo much

Source: Wikipedia

If you believe that this book is worth sharing, would you please take the time to let others know how it affected your life? If it turns out to make a difference in the lives of others, they will be forever grateful to you, as will I.

www.ingramcontent.com/pod-product-compliance
Lightning Source LLC
Chambersburg PA
CBHW060418290526
45791CB00002B/804